THE ARTHUR MURRAYS'

Dance Secrets

DRAWINGS BY OLGA LEY

New York, 1946

Dancing is "conversation" to music! When you dance, you express yourself. You hold your partner's interest through the correct use of musical rhythm, just as in good conversation you hold another's interest through use of the spoken word.

★ *Contents* ★

Arthur Murray

By His Wife

My husband is a two-faced man! At home, he is easy-going and amiable . . . he tells me that my cake is marvelous—even when it gives him indigestion.

But at the studio, he's a stickler for perfection . . . maintains that a teacher has no right to ever stop learning. He and the 200 instructors on our New York staff train forever!

He has a high regard for the value of good dancing. Perhaps this is because he was a very bashful boy— and dancing brought him friends and happiness. He is deeply satisfied when he can help someone who is shy and awkward to become graceful and self-confident; when he can see a lonely man or girl become popular and happy.

I am awed when I realize that over 3,000,000 people have learned to dance in my husband's schools . . . I am proud to find "Arthur Murray" in Who's Who and in the Encyclopaedia Britannica . . . and to know that his books are in every public library. But, although I am impressed—the man who has earned this reputation takes it for granted. He is genuinely amazed when teen-agers ask him for his autograph.

This won't be a surprise to you—but it's a daily thrill to me . . . Arthur Murray is a marvelous dancer!

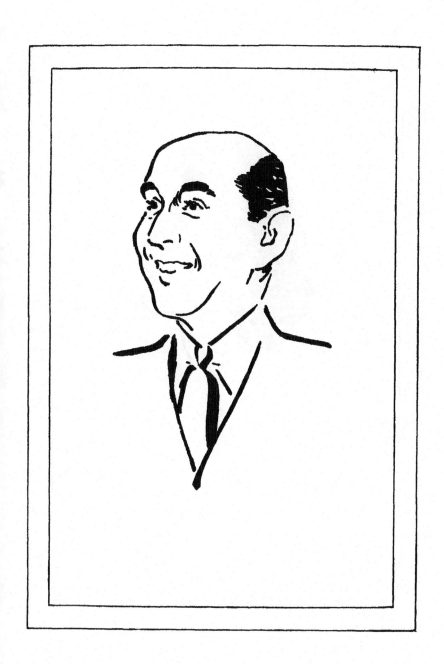

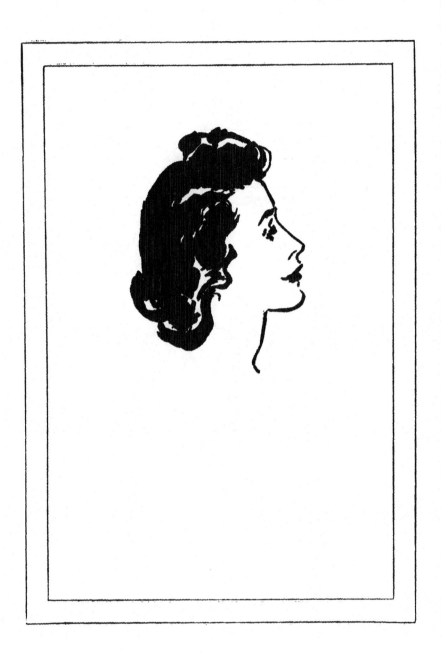

10

Kathryn Murray

By Her Husband

Mrs. Murray was a school-teacher before I married her. So quite naturally, after I had completed the manuscript for "Arthur Murray's Dance Secrets" and was about to send it to the printer, I asked her to look it over for grammatical errors.

Half an hour later Mrs. Murray turned to me and said: "Do you mind if I rewrite the first page?" A little later she said, "The second page seems too heavy-handed . . . do you mind if I rewrite that one, too?" After that she didn't ask for my permission to rewrite any other pages; she just sat at the typewriter and did not stop typing until she reached page 112. I then threw my own manuscript into the wastebasket!

I am glad to be married to Mrs. Murray . . . not because she writes so well or because she is the best cake baker in America . . . but because she does everything so much better than I do that I don't have to work any more.

It is nice to be able to drift into the office about one o'clock and spend the whole afternoon dancing, knowing that the management of the New York Studio and the 70 branches are in her small but capable hands.

Good Dancers Are Popular!

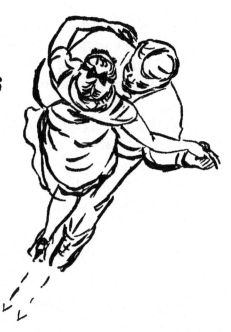

STOP and think a moment—do you know anyone who is a good dancer and who is not outstandingly popular? I doubt that you do. And that is the main reason why people want to be good dancers. There is nothing so thrilling in life as to be popular with friends and sought after as a companion.

It's Fun To Dance

It's easy to understand why good dancers are in demand. Just watch any crowd on a ballroom floor. Those who can dance well look happy—they seem in tune with the gaiety and music. Not only are they enjoying themselves, but their partners are having a fine time, too. People like to dance—they are born with a deep and inherent love of moving to rhythm.

There's nothing new about dancing—it is as old as mankind. Dancing used to have a serious side back in the dark ages. Primitive man had a different dance for every phase of emotion . . . his religion, superstition, grief, hate, happiness and love. Dancing has lived in every age, every class of life. High school students are always amused when they study the life of Socrates, the ancient philosopher—they can hardly believe their eyes when they read that he danced, too!

Physical Benefits of Dancing

We dance because it's fun—that's reason enough. But, dancing is also an easy, delightful form of exercise. Good dancers develop supple grace and superb muscle tone by using the muscles of the diaphragm, arms, shoulders, legs and ankles. Dancing is closely related to rhythmic sports such as tennis, skating and boxing.

Why Doctors Prescribe Dancing

Because dancing is so easy to learn and such a relaxing exercise, doctors prescribe it for many types of patients. A shy, awkward adolescent can become a graceful, well poised youth once he becomes confident of himself as a dancer. Middle-aged people who have slumped, given up and "let themselves go" can gain a new, vigorous, youthful posture and personality through a re-awakened interest in dancing. Certain physical defects can be improved and corrected by dancing

14

. . . it is used toward attaining better posture; strengthening weak arches and developing strong, graceful legs.

Dancing Lasts a Lifetime!

Now and then I have heard pupils complain of the "routine" involved in learning. Basic fundamentals are necessary in the beginning—just as you must learn to hold a golf club or a tennis racquet before you can play. But, once you have really learned to dance, it becomes something you will never forget. We often see white-haired couples doing a beautiful Waltz, just as proficiently as they did years ago. No matter how old a person is he can still move with youthful grace on the dance floor. Isn't it worth the effort of mastering the fundamentals to gain a lifetime of pleasure?

Don't Envy Others

I have never met any normal person who could not learn to become a fine dancer. You have the same natural ability that others have and good dancing is within your reach. Make up your mind today not to lose out on pleasure. Be a good dancer—have more fun out of life!

HOW TO WALK CORRECTLY
IN DANCING

There is never any reason to fear that you and your partner may falter or stumble at the beginning of a dance. Simply remember that a man *always* starts with his left foot . . . the girl, facing him, starts with her right foot.

Most men start each dance by walking forward, left foot first. So girls can be prepared and ready to walk backward, right foot first.

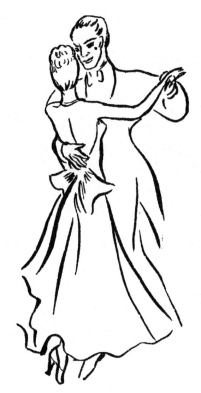

When You Dance:

Lift your feet slightly off the floor in all walking steps. Never let them scrape or drag on the floor.

★

When you walk backward, never let your heels touch the floor at all. When you walk forward, your heels may touch—but only after your toes have touched the floor first.

★

While you are learning, practice by walking only on the ball of the foot. You must emphasize this at the start . . . then, when you become proficient, your natural walking steps will be graceful, light and comfortable.

★

Emphasize and exaggerate only during your practice. When dancing with a partner, walk naturally without conscious strain or effort.

★

To give spring to your walking steps, practice rising up and down on your toes while taking long, slow walking steps around the room.

Secrets

That Will Help a Girl Become a Good Dancer

★ Convince yourself that the way to be light is to first strengthen the muscles you use in dancing. Watch an athlete walk across a floor . . . then watch someone who sits at a desk all day and whose muscles are slack. Which person walks lightly? *(Study the Exercises in this book)*

★ Prove to yourself that a girl must know the basic steps. Which of your girl friends are better dancers . . . those who know steps and can lead them or those who "don't know one step from another"?

★ Study this fact . . . a girl can follow only the steps that are familiar to her. Learn a VARIETY of steps so your partners won't be held back by you. Variety will put spice in your dancing!

★ Always remember: If you can dance well alone, you can then dance more easily and successfully with a partner. Practice in private—to be popular in public!

18

☆ Remember . . . a man is used to stepping forward—a girl must step backward most of the time!

☆ Stepping backward is not a natural motion—it must be practiced. But, once a girl can step back properly, her feet will never be in her partner's way. Besides, a girl cannot look graceful until she does master a long, free back step.

☆ A girl always starts with her right foot. Be ready! Practice your back walk alone, starting with your right foot and reaching far back *with your toes.*

☆ Take extremely long steps during your practice work. Stretch from your ankle with every step you take. Exaggerate when you are alone—then a normally long step will become second nature to you.

☆ Don't believe for a minute that you can "get by" by simply following a partner. Thousands of girls make this mistake—but none of the popular girls do. Decide now to spend a little time and effort to become the kind of dancer you'd like to be. You can do it—make up your mind to try!

Remember: Confidence comes only with knowledge. Your partner, too, will have confidence in you if you are sure of yourself.

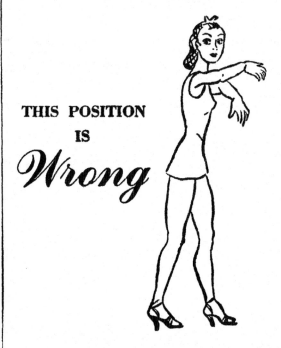

THIS POSITION
IS
Wrong

It is absolutely impossible for a girl to dance well when her feet are placed flat on the floor. In this position her steps will be short . . . and her partner will be unable to strike out with a long, free, easy dancing stride.

Not only will she be a heavy handicap to her partner, but her feet will appear large and clumsy on the floor.

20

THIS POSITION
IS
Right

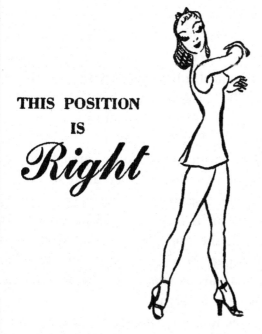

Note that when the toes lead, a girl's step becomes long and free moving . . . and that her foot looks graceful.

Here is an easy trick—imagine that you want to point the way in every step with your one big toe —let it lead whichever way you move.

REACH WITH THE TOE; stretching from the ankle —not from the hip.

21

★ *Why Girls Too Must Know The Steps* ★

WHENEVER I hear a woman say: "All I need is a good leader" . . . I know that she is probably a poor dancer and that partners steer clear of her.

"Leading" must be a misleading word—so many girls confuse it with "dragging"! The leader is merely the one who chooses the steps and guides his partner into them. But, unless his partner is *alert* and ready to dance with him, she becomes a tag-along, an extra weight to be carried around.

A girl cannot dance *with* her partner until she knows what she is doing. She can test her own knowledge by trying to dance alone to music or by leading a girl partner. If she feels helpless by herself, she can tell immediately that she does not know her own part. It will be safer for her to refuse invitations until she has learned what she needs to make her popular and fun to have as a partner.

Once a girl becomes interested in the steps themselves, she will enjoy learning. She will begin to notice dancing technique on the stage, the screen and among her friends. Only a good dancer knows the thrill of accomplishment . . . poor dancers don't know what they are missing. The more steps a girl knows, the more spontaneity she will show in her dancing.

A girl who is *not animated* strikes a negative response. Partners do not return willingly to her and social evenings are a gamble . . . will she be popular or not? It is a pity for a girl to take a chance when a little effort can make her confident and sure. A girl who can do the steps alone will never be left alone at a dance.

22

You Can Learn
to Keep Time!

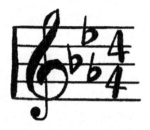

PEOPLE sometimes like to brag about their deficiencies. They will say, proudly: "I have terrible handwriting" ... or ... "I have no memory—I can never think of a person's name." In the studio, we often hear this said: "But, I can't carry a tune on a bet!"

The ability to carry a tune is not a necessary factor in learning to dance. To dance, you must simply be able to keep time to the music. And if you can march to band music— you can keep time to dance music.

The unfortunate belief that they have "no sense of rhythm" keeps many people from enjoying the pleasures of

23

dancing. Yet, every normal person is born with a sense of rhythm. In some cases, it may need developing but it's there. Forget about the idea that you must have a knowledge of music—nine out of ten good dancers don't know one note from another, yet they can keep time.

If You Can't Carry a Tune

REMEMBER this, dancers do not keep time to the melody or the tune of a song. The high and low notes have nothing to do with it. The count in dancing is determined by the *beat* or tempo of the music.

So, if you can't sing, hum or whistle a simple tune like "Yankee Doodle," don't despair. It won't keep you from becoming a good dancer, although it should keep you from singing in your partner's ear!

Here are two simple ways to train yourself to keep time:

1. Beat time with your foot.

2. Walk in time to Fox Trot music.

24

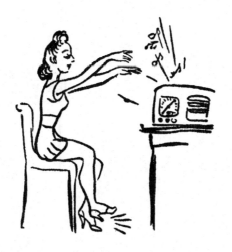

1

Sit next to your radio or victrola and listen to any dance music. Imagine that you are the drummer and simply beat time with your foot on the floor as though you were hitting the pedal of the bass drum. Tap your hand on the chair arm at the same time. Keep tapping to different types of music until it becomes automatic to follow the drum beat.

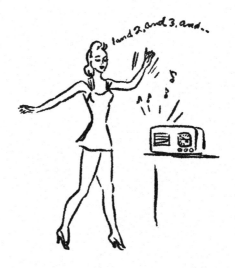

2

After you have learned to beat time, walk around the room, taking one step to each beat. Do this in private, so that you will not feel self-conscious. Try walking to several different songs. In a surprisingly short while, your feet will "carry the tune" easily.

And that's all there is to keeping time to music!

How to Hold Your Partner

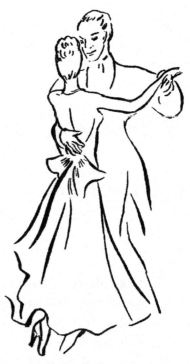

THERE is nothing mysterious about "how to hold your partner" in dancing. Your position should be guided by comfort, common sense and convention—and that is all there is to it.

Outside of a few eccentric crazes like the Bunny Hug, Charleston, Black Bottom and so on, position in ballroom dancing hasn't changed appreciably in the past 30 years.

Youngsters have always had fads in their dancing style. One year you may find young girls leaving their right arms outstretched, palms up—as though feeling for raindrops. By the next season they will have forgotten that fad and will adopt another distinctive style.

Some youngsters assume exaggerated dancing positions

27

merely to cover their embarrassment at not knowing what to do. As their dancing improves, they will drop affectations. Young people are more comfortable when they dance exactly as their friends do—wise parents realize this and overlook short-lived styles.

In this book we are concerned only with presenting to you the quickest and easiest means of becoming a good dancer—popular with all partners. A correct dancing position will help to make this possible.

1 You can practice correct dancing position very easily in your own room, without a partner. Face a mirror and stand erect. Don't strain—simply stand naturally and comfortably as though you were about to walk down the street. Now rise so that your weight is placed evenly on the soles of your shoes —no weight on your heels. Hum a popular tune and walk about in time to the rhythm until you feel fully at ease.

2 You will find it helpful to raise your arms in typical dancing position as you practice alone. Do not hold your elbows unnaturally high—it is tiring, unnecessary and out-of-date. Glance in the mirror and you will see that a medium elbow-height forms the most graceful line.

3 Looking at yourself standing erect, with your arms up, will remind you to hold yourself tall. Good dancing posture is

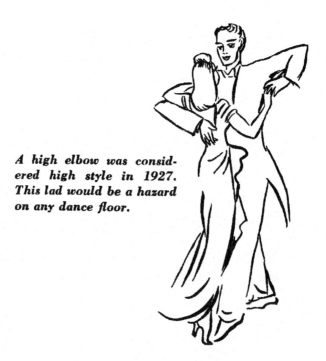

A high elbow was considered high style in 1927. This lad would be a hazard on any dance floor.

flattering. It will help you to form the habit of holding your head high, with your chest out and chin in. Bring out the best in your looks!

4 Remember to keep your heels off the floor as much as possible. A flat-footed, firm stance belongs on the golf course —not on the dance floor. Keeping your weight over the soles of your feet will make you feel quicker and lighter as a partner.

5 Here is one of the most important things for you to remember. Without this, you can never hope to be a good dancer or to even "get by" in appearance. Keep your feet

29

close together, unless you are taking a definite step to the side. Walk toward your mirror in dance position . . . see how you look when your feet are apart. It's not a pretty sight, is it? Now, walk again and make a conscious effort to pass your feet closely together. Are you sold on why this is so important in dancing?

6 For graceful dancing, you must learn to turn your toes out, rather than in. Again, a peek at your mirror will convince you why this looks better.

7 Now is the time for you to stop worrying. You have seen yourself as others will see you, so you should feel secure and

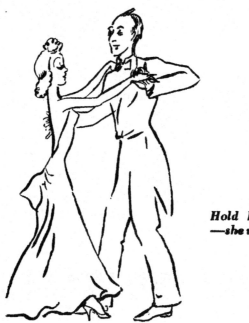

*Hold her closer
—she won't bite!*

CULTIVATE LIGHTNESS

It is vital. Practicing the basic steps in dancing—*especially practicing them alone*—is the first trick in learning lightness.

Once the basic steps have become second nature with you, learn a variety of steps. You can follow —or lead—only as many steps as you know well. Make sure you do not sacrifice perfection for variety.

ready for teamwork with a partner. When dancing with someone, adopt the position that is most comfortable for both of you. Not so close together that you have no freedom of movement—but not too far apart.

8 Do not curl your arm under your partner's. Fancy, trick holds should be put away with your high school diploma.

9 A man leads best when he hold his partner in front of him or an inch or so to his right . . . no tape measure necessary . . . we're dancing for fun!

10 Easy does it. Don't plan to lean forward or backward— just assume a natural, comfortable position and your partner will find you a natural, comfortable dancing companion.

HOW TO HOLD YOUR PARTNER

Hints for the Man

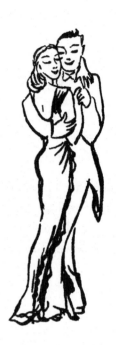

This is an interesting way to hold your partner—but not on the dance floor. A couple wrapped up in themselves make a silly looking package to the onlookers.

● There is a logical reason for a man's left arm to be extended while he dances. It is held out so as to avoid collisions with other couples as you dance by. But, your arm does not have to extend as rigidly and inflexibly as a bumper—nor does your elbow have to be held at an uncomfortably sharp angle. Simply hold the girl's hand lightly but firmly, with your left arm in an easy, graceful curve.

● As you dance, look over the girl's right shoulder. By holding your partner directly in front of you or a bit to your right, you will have a clear view of what's ahead. You are the leader—so it is up to you to choose a clear path.

● Hold your partner firmly enough to guide her. A weak, listless hold will not inspire her confidence in you. Hold your

32

hand at a comfortable height on the middle of her back. There is no cut-and-dried rule for this . . . although a doctor once did stump me by asking: "Which vertebra shall I hold?"

● Always start your first step forward with your left foot. Let your toes lead and step directly toward your partner's right foot. Don't worry, she'll be moving hers backward.

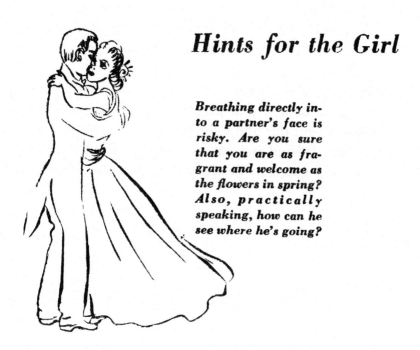

Hints for the Girl

Breathing directly into a partner's face is risky. Are you sure that you are as fragrant and welcome as the flowers in spring? Also, practically speaking, how can he see where he's going?

● As you dance, look over your partner's right shoulder for two reasons:

1. Your feet naturally point in the same direction as your eyes. By looking ahead, you will stay in correct and comfortable alignment with your partner.

2. It may seem fascinating at first but it soon becomes an uncomfortable strain when partners gaze hypnotically at each other while dancing. Try it with a girl friend . . . you'll find that she looks owl-like when her face is too close to yours.

● Always be ready to take your first step backward with your right foot. A man steps forward on his left . . . give him a chance to get going.

● Let your toes lead in every step that you take. It will lengthen your step by at least six inches. Besides, stretching out with your toes, will make you look ten times better to the stag line.

● The secret of good balance is to hold your left hand very firmly on the back of your partner's right shoulder. You will find more about this under the pointers on following. Never wrap your left hand and arm around your partner's neck . . . it won't add glamour—it will simply pull you off balance.

How to Judge Character by Dancing

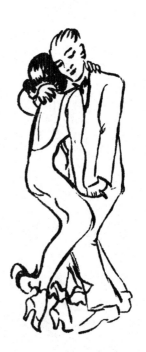

the cuddly couple

WANT to play a new game on "How To Judge Character"? Just watch 'em dance—they give themselves away. Here are some clues to get you started . . .

There are those who love themselves—can you spot them? They point their toes too gracefully and meticulously, stepping very carefully indeed. And why shouldn't they take good care of the ten little tootsies that are THEIRS!

The "cuddly couples" are fun to watch—unless you're related to them! Dance floor petters never outgrow the urge. You can put bells on their toes and wedding rings on their fingers—they'll still cuddle!

Here's one of masculine gender only. He meanders around the floor, pushing his partner into everything that

35

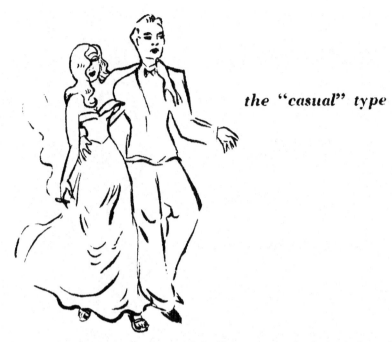

the "casual" type

comes his way. He's inconsiderate and thoughtless. Marry his type and life will be one traffic jam after another—with you as the bumper!

Then there are the "casual" ones. The girl, with sloppy "I-don't-care" posture and the man, jes' shufflin' along. She's probably a job-drifter hoping for the divine job with hours from 12 to 1 . . . and with an hour off for lunch. When she marries, she'll be a handy gal with a can opener. And her limping hazard? The world owes him a living—you might as well deliver it right to his door. Oh—and on the way in— please pick up the socks he dropped the night before.

Know the brand marks of jealousy? The possessive man cups his hand tightly on his partner's back. His posture is

36

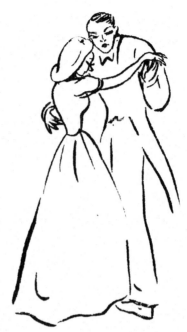

the timid souls

crouching, as though ready for a springing pounce. If your heart belongs to that Daddy, then throw in your body and soul, too. He's a mine-all-mine lad. . . . Now the trouble with a jealous gal is that her little ways are so fetching—at first. She clings to her partner's arm like glue, looks up in his eyes with an "Aren't you wonderful" effect and is so attentive that she goes to his head. But, her husband will have a male secretary if she has anything to say!

Don't look too hard for the timid souls—they'll sink to the floor if you stare at them. The masculine variety has low slung elbows, an apologetic manner and a hang-dog expression. He takes faltering steps and barely touches his partner. He's hard to follow because he's too shy to lead. . . . The girls of this type take uncertain steps, droop their arms and get an until-death-do-us-part grip on their partner's left thumb. *(Are you a timid soul?)*

Beware of the bully—you can spot him on sight. He swings his partner around fast and furiously, with complete disregard for her clothes, hair and general well-being. He turns his toes outward, showing that he is vain as well as self-indulgent. Thumbs down on him if that's how he dances!

The show-off can't be so bad—his mother loves him! But, look out when he holds his elbows high . . . he shows arrogance and vanity. Besides, he may knock your eye out!

It takes all kinds to make a world—and you'll find one of each on every dance floor. Watch their steps!

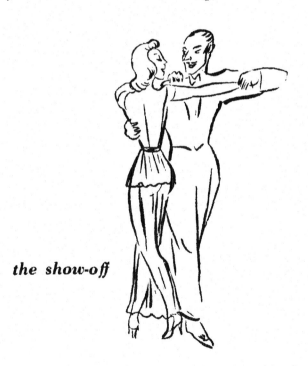

the show-off

The Secrets of Leading

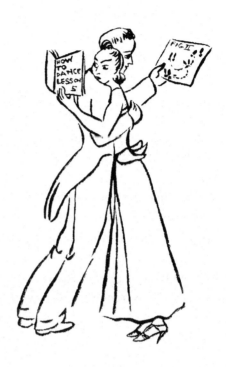

THE dance floor is the one place where the weaker sex prefers to remain submissive. Girls expect their partners to set the pace—to choose and direct the steps. All that they ask of you is a definite indication of where you are heading.

To give this definite indication, a man must first be clearly certain of just what he does want to do. If he is not sure of himself, how can he expect a partner to be able to follow him? There is no short-cut to good leading ... it takes a definite, well defined knowledge of the steps.

So, the one and only rule is ... KNOW THE STEPS! Then you will move with assurance and your partners will feel a glow of pride and confidence in your ability. You'll enjoy overhearing them say: "Isn't he a wonderful leader!"

Forceful Guiding Unnecessary

Believe it or not, the little woman does not need to be pushed, pulled or hauled to make her go your way. When you can do your own part well, you won't have to worry about leading. Reserve your strong-arm tactics for other times, other places than the dance floor.

Sometimes, when dancing with a brand new partner who can follow but is not yet familiar with your style of dancing, you may have to do a bit of guiding. This is done with your right hand and arm. Always hold your right hand firmly just above your partner's waist—you will find that she will re-

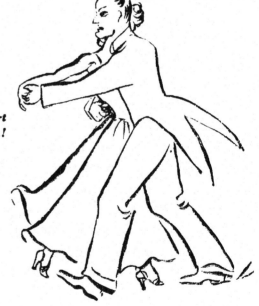

Wrestling is a manly art
—keep it for the men!

spond easily to a light pressure. Your left hand does very little toward leading.

Pointers for Good Leaders

● When dancing with a new partner for the first time, start off with very simple steps. You then become acquainted with each other's style in dancing.

● Simple, uninvolved steps are easy to lead and follow and they will quickly give you and your partner ease and confidence in each other. There is plenty of time ahead for your more advanced, intricate steps and turns.

● Most good dancers lead the same step at least twice in succession . . . it makes their dancing more flowing—and it gives them time to plan a graceful sequence to their pattern of steps. It is far better to do the same step several times than rush into quick, jerky changes.

● Don't be afraid to pause, in position with your partner, at the beginning of each dance. Listen to the music, make sure of your timing and then start forward, sure and confident of yourself.

● Never count for your partner unless you don't care what she thinks of you. Neither is it necessary for you to tell her, in words, what you expect to do next. Knowing your own part well and holding your right hand firmly on her back will convey a sufficient message to her.

41

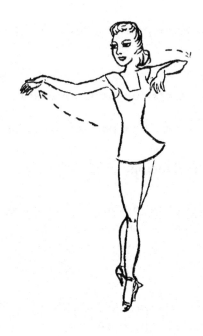

Which is a Right Turn?

To make a right turn, look over your right shoulder and let the rest of your body follow.
To make a right turn, move the left hand forward.

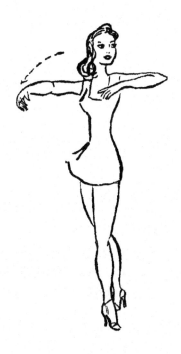

—and Which is a Left?

To make a left turn, look over your left shoulder and let the rest of your body follow.

To make a left turn, move the left hand backward.

To be a really good dancer, you must be able to dance without having to concentrate on your steps. Your feet must have learned to respond easily to the music; you must be able to lead or follow without apparent effort.

How
Learning to Lead
Will Help
A Girl's Dancing

IF YOU are like most girls and women, you will be shocked when you read this . . . "To be a better dancer, learn to lead!"

But, here's a simple test that may help to convince you. Think back to the girls you knew at school. Select those girls who were in demand at every dance—the girls who had plenty of "cut-ins," who were never wallflowers. Now, think it over . . . weren't they the ones who could lead the other girls as partners?

I first hit upon this theory many years ago. The idea of teaching girls to lead was completely contrary to the accepted beliefs of the day. However, I was sure of the logic and common sense in back of my theory and I decided to try it out.

I visited classes that we held in girls' clubs, schools and colleges. I asked the members of each group to vote for the best dancers among their girl friends. Without a single exception, every good dancer who was selected was a girl who could lead!

Frankly, it has taken a great deal of courage to uphold my strong convictions. Most women cling tenaciously to the belief that "Leading will ruin a girl's dancing." It usually takes me a long time to convince mothers that their daughters can become popular dancing partners more quickly by first learning to lead other girls.

The Arthur Murray girl teachers are noted for their ability to follow any partner. The first step in their training is to learn to lead all partners in all dances. In our studios we now teach all girl pupils to lead before teaching them to follow.

Two Reasons Why Learning to Lead Will Make a Girl a Better Dancer

1 Have you ever skated hand-in-hand? If so, you know that it is only fun when you and your partner strike out and glide at the same moment. If one of you is slower and misses the rhythm, two-some skating becomes boring and uncomfortable.

Dancing with a partner works on the same principle. A girl must dance *with* her partner—not *after* him. She must express herself in time with the music . . . not wait woodenly and lifelessly, dependent on a strong push-and-pull lead. A

46

girl who can lead understands the music and she can step out rhythmically, at the exact same time as her partner. Any man will enjoy her dancing because it feels alert—alive—vital.

2 Once a girl can lead, she begins to realize and appreciate the man's part. She discovers what she is expected to do when she is following a partner. A girl who can lead the man's part in any step, will be able to follow that step twice as lightly and twice as well. To dance with true poise and assurance, you need the confidence that knowledge brings. Learn to lead each step first . . . then you'll follow it like a breeze.

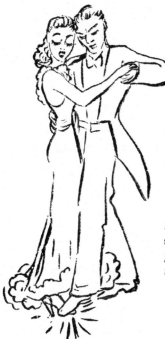

If she could lead, her feet would move WITH her partner's . . . not after, or under his!

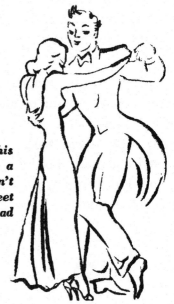

Even a trick twist like this would be no mystery to a girl who can lead. Don't study your partner's feet . . . study his part—ahead of time.

Exceptions to Girls' Leading

In all fairness to the old-fashioned prejudice against girls leading, there are certain exceptions to the rule. But, it is only in these two cases that leading will be a drawback to a girl's dancing.

● A girl should not lead other girls more than half the time. The two girls should take equal turns. Sometimes tall girls are forced into leading too often merely because of their height. They should single out other tall girls with whom to practice.

48

On the other hand, short girls should not forego the benefits of leading simply because their friends tower above them. It is a bit harder to lead someone much taller than yourself . . . but it is not really difficult; it will seem easy with practice. A short man dislikes dancing with a tall girl—not because it is difficult—but because he is afraid that the difference in size will make him look comic. A short girl has nothing to fear on this score . . . she should feel confident of being able to lead any girl partner.

● Note that the following exception to the rule of girls leading applies only to poor dancers.

A girl will gain nothing from leading if she leads the same few steps all of the time. Her muscles will become accustomed to only these few movements and habit will force her into the same steps no matter how strongly her partner leads. She will be in a rut and she will feel stiff and heavy to a man partner.

To gain the full value from leading, a girl must practice leading as many steps as she hopes to be able to follow.

If you have any personal dance problems, please do not hesitate to write, telephone or visit your nearest Arthur Murray Studio for aid. Our teachers will be glad to demonstrate any of the steps taught in this book. See list of studios on last page.

How to Follow

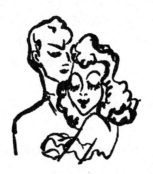

I ONCE met a girl who was very unhappy. She said to me: "I don't understand it, Mr. Murray, boys never cut-in on me but I know I can dance — why, I can follow anyone." I danced with her and found that she could follow, provided that I led her in the few simple steps with which she was familiar. As soon as I attempted anything more advanced, she was at a complete loss.

I asked her: "Do most of your partners do these same steps I've been doing with you?" "Why yes," she said. "That's exactly the way they dance."

So I explained that her partners were held down — they could do only those few steps because those were all she could follow. I showed her that I could not lead her in any of my other steps without having her falter or stumble.

That girl is only one of the many girls and women who

believe that they can follow anyone . . . and then they wonder why they are not in demand as partners.

A man is limited in his dancing to what his partner can do. He finds it dull and uninteresting when he is hampered in his choice of steps—and bound down by his partner's lack of knowledge. Here is a list of pointers that will help you to become a popular dancer, sought-after over and over again. Note that the very first essential is in Rule 1.

10 Rules For Following

1 Know the basic steps and their possible combinations. Isn't it logical that you cannot dance well with a man until you are familiar with the steps he will do?

2 Next, give your partner a feeling of freedom in his forward steps—keep your feet out of his way. You can develop a long, free, swinging backward step. Try it . . . step back as far as possible, toes leading. Keep your foot off the floor until you step with your weight on it. Exaggerate by lifting your feet high off the floor as you practice.

3 Let your toes lead! Look at your foot when you take a plain walking step. Now watch what happens when you stretch with your toes. It is a simple matter of arithmetic . . . you can add actual inches to your step by merely pointing your

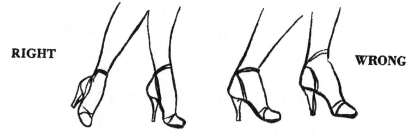

RIGHT   WRONG

Let your toes point the way to good dancing.

toes. Practice a long, graceful stride backward, forward and to each side—letting your big toe point the way.

4 Here's another foot-note . . . practice dancing on your toes—it will help to make you lighter.

5 Be ready for the next step—come what may. Want to know how? Don't slide your feet along the floor—lift and pass them through the air instead. Invest in practicing this . . . it pays big dividends in popularity with partners.

6 A short step may seem dainty to you but it will spell disaster to your dancing. Prove this to yourself by leading one of your girl friends. Tell her to take short steps—it will convince you immediately why you need to develop a long dancing stride.

7 Track down the true meaning of the word "relax." Try

53

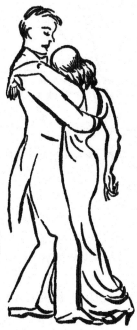

Relaxing completely makes a girl as heavy as lead to lead!

relaxing while you stand in front of a mirror. Do you look like a dancer, full of life and spirit? You can bet you don't! When you relax, your body sags—if you were with a partner, your full weight would drop on him. Dancing is motion—pep it up!

8 The opposite of complete relaxation is "tenseness." But, you cannot cure a stiff, tense body by commanding it to relax. Tenseness comes from a feeling of insecurity and from a lack of training. Learning the steps will give you security and confidence . . . practicing the "Exercises" in this book will give you training. Don't envy popular girls—rival them!

9 This should have a page to itself—so don't overlook it. It is the answer on how to have good balance. No girl can be a pleasure to lead until she can balance her own weight. It's a pity that so few girls know that their balance is in their own hands!

Simply hold firmly with your left hand just in back of your partner's right shoulder. Hold on very firmly—he won't feel your weight, I promise you.

10 Learn your steps and train your muscles on your own time. Then you will be automatically limber and ready to follow a partner—without a thought of your feet or your steps. He's the leader . . . don't be ahead of him or drag after him—just dance *with* him.

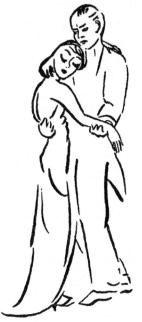

A dream girl becomes a nightmare when she's heavy. Hold yourself up!

To be a Good Dancer —

Keep your feet out of your partner's way. Develop a long, free, swinging step by stretching your toes backward. The easy, graceful step is taken by leading with the big toe. backward.

Move naturally, easily, comfortably. Don't be self-conscious or stiff. Don't think the other couples are watching you. They're probably concentrating on themselves and each other.

56

How Tall Girls Can Appear Smaller

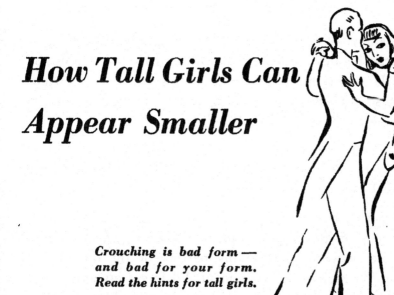

*Crouching is bad form —
and bad for your form.
Read the hints for tall girls.*

ONE characteristic that is admired in American girls is their height and fine bearing. Whereas most short girls yearn to be taller—few tall girls would trade places with them. Tall girls should be proud of their size . . . they should remember that models, who are selected for beauty of appearance, are always well above average height.

However, short men do avoid dancing with girls who tower above them. They are afraid of looking insignificant and comic—even when they secretly admire the girl's appearance.

Tall girls can be smart—they can seem shorter to partners

57

whenever they choose. Here are two pointers that work:

● KEEP YOUR ELBOWS LOW when you dance. You will appear shorter because your partners will not have to reach upward for dancing position. But, practice this with your girl friends first so you can avoid resting your arms heavily on your partner.

● Without changing your natural standing posture in any way, LET YOUR KNEES BEND SLIGHTLY. This will reduce your height by several inches. Practice in private!

Perhaps you will feel that these suggestions do not enhance your appearance. But, if I were a girl, and had to choose between pleasing my partner or the onlookers, I wouldn't hesitate for a moment. I'd forget my appearance, if need be, and stand so that my partner would feel comfortable and would want to dance with me again.

Bent knees, by the way, will not show with long skirts.

Dangers for Tall Girls to Avoid

Tall girls should never try to appear smaller by leaning forward. This will make you difficult to lead, whether your partner is tall or short. Your hips and feet will be too far apart from your partner's and you will not only look, but feel awkward in all steps. It is an impossible position in which to follow turning steps.

Do not take short steps. No matter how tall you are, you can never take too long a step ... don't worry—your partner's right hand will act as a safety brake.

Be proud of your height—and carry it proudly!

Six Helpful Hints
for Little Girls

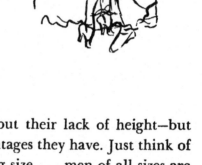

Little girls add inches to their height when they dance on the tips of their toes.

Little girls often complain about their lack of height—but they never remember the advantages they have. Just think of it—no partner is ever the wrong size . . . men of all sizes are possible partners.

Even the smallest girl, whose vision is bounded by vest buttons, can be a comfortable, adjustable partner to a six-foot-plus. Here are confidential hints to pint-sizers:

1 Train yourself to dance on the tips of your toes instead of balancing your weight on the soles of your feet. Practice this, at home and alone, until you can stretch and reach smoothly.

59

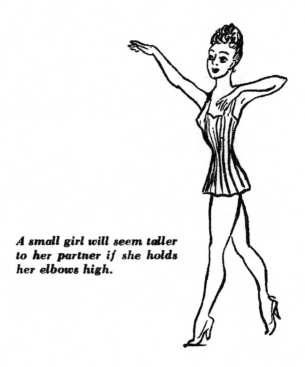

A small girl will seem taller to her partner if she holds her elbows high.

2 Always imagine that you are trying to touch the ceiling with the top of your head. Stretch high up, from the waist, to gain height.

3 Here is the most valuable tip of all . . . LEAD WITH YOUR TOES! You can actually see in your mirror that by reaching back, with your big toe leading, that you have lengthened your step from four to six inches. By doing this, your steps will be as long as those taken by a girl five inches taller than you are! Happy now?

60

4 Hold your elbows as high as you can. Practice alone, holding your arms bent in partner position—as high up as possible. Exaggerate . . . and your muscles will be strengthened and ready for the real thing.

5 Always hold firmly with your left hand at the back of your partner's shoulder. No matter how hard you grip—it will be welcome to him. All men find it easier to lead a girl who holds firmly to their right shoulders.

6 Never take short steps. Practice until you can step forward, backward and to each side with a long, graceful stride. (Toes leading.)

Just to cheer you up—many of our famous exhibition dancers aren't over 5 feet 2.

DON'TS
for Beginners

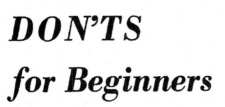
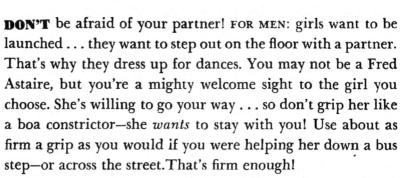

Hold that line! . . . But, hold it straight. Dance in upright position—same as while walking. You don't have to hoist the lady—just hold her.

DON'T be afraid of your partner! FOR MEN: girls want to be launched . . . they want to step out on the floor with a partner. That's why they dress up for dances. You may not be a Fred Astaire, but you're a mighty welcome sight to the girl you choose. She's willing to go your way . . . so don't grip her like a boa constrictor—she *wants* to stay with you! Use about as firm a grip as you would if you were helping her down a bus step—or across the street. That's firm enough!

FOR GIRLS: Don't grip him so hard that he thinks he's your last chance. There is only one spot for a strong hold . . .

62

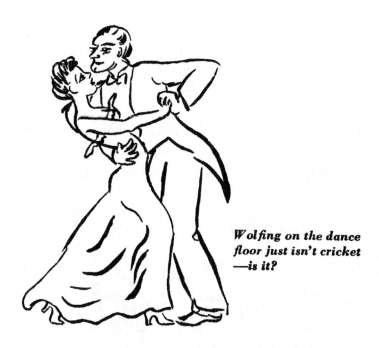

Wolfing on the dance floor just isn't cricket —is it?

and that is to take a firm grip, with your left hand, on the back of his right shoulder.

DON'T worry, if you're the leader, about how you will get in step with the music. All good dancers pause, in dance position, at the beginning. They listen to the tempo before they start. There is no law that says you must start with the very first note that the orchestra plays. Listen first. Remember that the distinctive rhythm of each type of music repeats itself every three or four seconds. You're bound to hear it.

Start off with your left foot on the accented—or heaviest—beat in the music. If you miss the first one, wait for the next. In Fox Trot, the first of every two beats is accented. In the Waltz, the first of every three beats is the most definite.

DON'T worry about the onlookers when you step out on the floor. The other dancers are too interested in themselves to pay attention to you and the "kibitzers" are too busy wishing they had partners. If you know your own part, you and your partner will feel well and look well . . . so, let yourself go straight ahead for fun and good times.

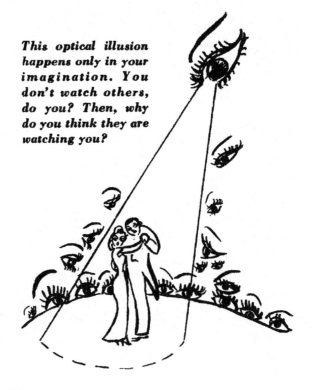

This optical illusion happens only in your imagination. You don't watch others, do you? Then, why do you think they are watching you?

How to be Graceful

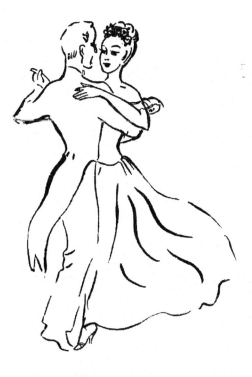

THIS IS NOT MEANT FOR GIRLS ONLY. Watch a tennis player, swimmer, skater—even a boxer—and you will realize that men can be graceful, too. To be graceful means to move lightly and without effort. We are not born with this ability; it comes only through training and strengthening the muscles.

When you train to gain muscular control, your movements must be exaggerated at the start. A football player, who wants to be able to kick a ball accurately, at the height of his waist, practices until he can kick as high as his head. Then the lower distance seems so easy that he can reach it with no effort at all.

Good dancers not only feel graceful to their partners but

they also look graceful in motion. Study and practice these pointers—they will help you to acquire a smooth, smart dancing appearance. Remember, exaggerate at the start and you will reach perfection with ease.

How To Use Your Feet Gracefully

● Lead with your toes when moving forward, backward and to the sides. Actually stretch from the ankle until your muscles can feel the pull. Dance about the room, practicing this motion.

● Keep your toes turned slightly outward. This is not a

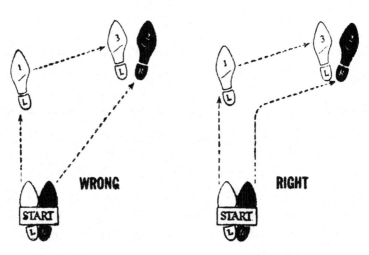

Remember this rule . . . Before taking a step to the side, always bring your feet together.

natural position; it will take conscious effort to acquire it.

● Your toes should always touch the floor first, whether you are dancing forward, backward or to the side. Avoid a flat-footed step!

● Always keep your feet as close together as the step permits. Even when your feet are moving in different directions, as in the illustrated footprints, you will note that they should pass closely—almost brushing against each other—rather than to be spread at an angle.

This secret of graceful footwork is important to you. Read the preceding paragraph again. Then study the footprints and try the step in front of your mirror. See how different it looks when your feet pass close together.

Graceful Body Motion

Body motion is governed entirely by the movement of your feet. In walking, when you step forward with your left foot, your right arm moves forward. You don't have to stop and think about it—it is automatic.

Therefore, don't attempt to acquire graceful body motion by consciously swaying from the waist. This won't work. Strive for graceful footwork and your body will naturally and easily move in a graceful dancing position.

How to Achieve
Perfect Carriage

IT IS annoying to be told to "stand up straight". Yet, we all envy the appearance of those with good posture. When a person wants to look his best, he automatically lifts his head and stands tall and erect. There is no trick to achieving perfect carriage—it's easy to learn. Then, once it becomes a habit, it is yours forever.

An army man needs no uniform to display his soldierly bearing. Through practice, he has developed fine posture. You can tell at a glance that he's an army man.

Dancing, like military training, accustoms the body to fall in line, without the necessity of effort or reminders. Very few people can train themselves to adopt good posture, by will power alone. If you walk along the street and think: "I must stand more erect"—you do so, but for a few moments only. As soon as you stop thinking about it, you slump back into your old ways.

But when you take up a new muscular activity, such as dancing, which constantly requires correct posture, you have the chance of a lifetime to replace old, faulty habits with new and good ones. It is a good idea to practice new dance steps in front of a mirror—your reflection will prompt you to adopt

"an army man"

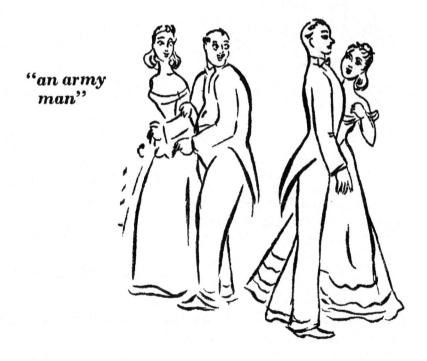

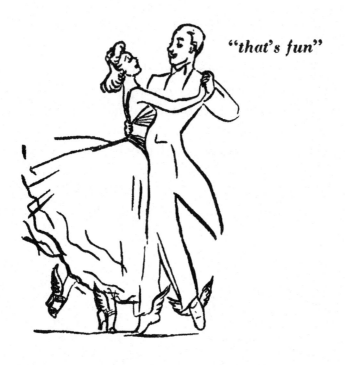

"that's fun"

an attractive and flattering position. Before you know it, good posture will come quite naturally to you.

★ ★ ★

Dancing needs soul—not soles. You have seen couples whose feet fairly fly. That's fun! If they can do it, you can, too. Practice will put wings on your feet.

Pumping your arms or flouncing your elbows betrays an unconscious attempt to keep time to the music because your feet can't do it. Train yourself to be nimble and quick— don't accept substitutes!

Swaying the body from the hips is fine for high school calisthenics. A good dancer moves from the hips down.

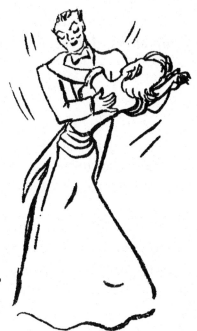

"from the hips down"

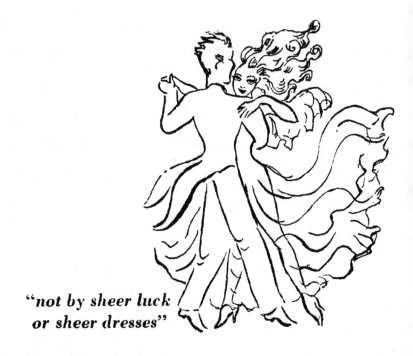

*"not by sheer luck
or sheer dresses"*

A rose by any other name would be just as lovely—provided it has an upright stem to show it off. To droop is to wilt . . . keep your head and shoulders UP.

Good dancers float through the air — but they do it through training and practice. It can't be done by sheer luck or sheer dresses. A smiling glance in your direction may mean amusement—not admiration.

Rising too high on your toes will make you look and

72

feel tense and stiff. Try walking around the room, perched unnaturally high on your toes—do you like the effect?

This is "for men only"! A girl dresses to suit you—not to be spread-eagled over your suit. Avoid deep dips and brusque or sudden motions. She's dressed for dancing, **not for wrestling.**

Do not bend your knees any more in dancing than in walking. A bent knee may make the wrong impression **on** your partner.

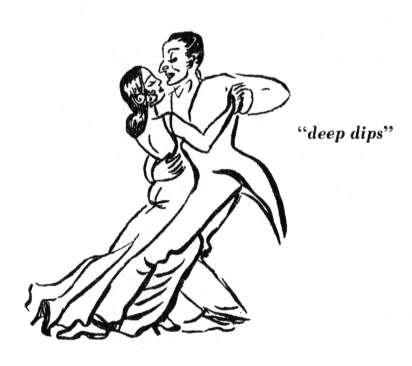

"deep dips"

Placing your feet apart will give you a firm stance in golf —but too firm a stand for dancing. Plant your feet in neat rows, close together, and you'll harvest a crop of admiration.

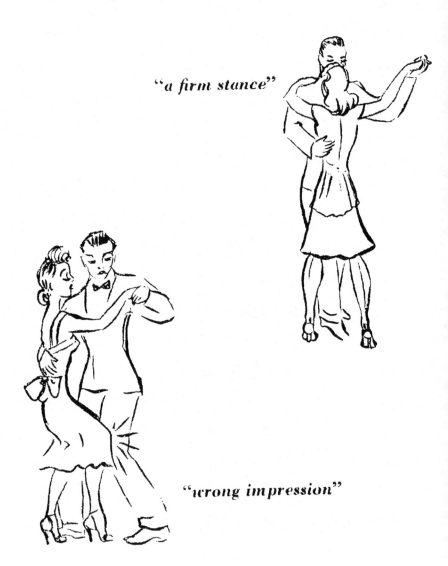

"a firm stance"

"wrong impression"

Heavy, heavy, hangs the partner who cannot lift feet from floor. If you drag along—or scrape—or hug the floor; you cannot float or glide. Practice new steps by exaggerating the lifting motion of your feet.

Above all, be natural. Remember that the other dancers are busy enjoying themselves, not looking to criticize you. Let yourself go with the music and your partner.

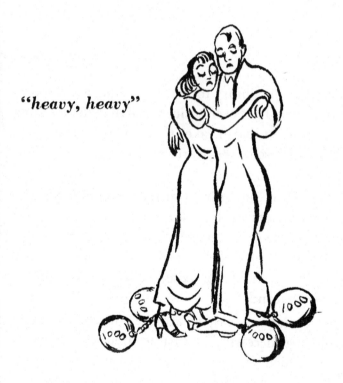

"heavy, heavy"

The Secret of Good Balance

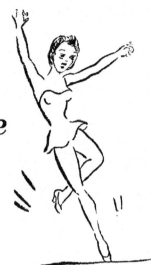

Good balance is the ability to maintain your equilibrium easily, lightly. If you have ever noticed a small child, toddling about, you have seen that it takes time before a steady, upright walk is achieved. We learn to balance our weight through practice.

Before we go on, supposing you try this simple balance test. Place your weight on the toes of one foot, raising the other foot off the floor for several inches, either forward or backward. Do you feel as steady as the Rock of Gibraltar? Most people cannot hold this pose, without wavering, for more than a few seconds.

But, good balance is easy to acquire. In dancing, there are just two things necessary . . . first, to strengthen the muscles of the toes which carry your weight—second, and for girls only, learn to use your left hand as ballast—to give you added support.

Both men and girls can improve their balance and strengthen their toe muscles by dancing alone and by practicing the exercises in this book. Many men feel self-confident— they are not afraid of being wallflowers because they know that they can always ask a girl to dance. But, if those men who "get by" with poor dancing could hear what their partners say about them in the Powder Room, they might be more anxious to improve their technique.

Strengthening the toe muscles will serve you well in other fields than dancing. Good balance is required for football, basketball, tennis, skating, boxing, track and golf. Further, good balance gives you an attractive and a tireless walking posture.

FOR GIRLS

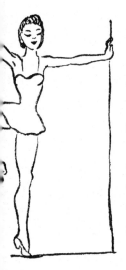

Try the "balance test" again; placing your weight on the toes of one foot, with the other foot extended in air. Now place your left hand on the top of your dresser or on the back of a chair. It's easy to stand steadily now, isn't it?

When you dance, train yourself to hold your left hand very firmly on the back of your partner's shoulder. Don't be afraid, you will not seem heavy. He will not feel the slightest discomfort from that pressure. Instead, you will seem lighter to him. If

77

you would like to prove this to yourself, lead one of your girl friends. Have her hold on to your shoulder, steadying her full weight with her left hand. You will find that you can lead her easily, even if she drops her right arm completely.

This is the first bit of training that I give to every girl teacher in our studios. My experience has been that I must repeat this warning several times to each girl . . . HOLD YOUR LEFT HAND FIRMLY ON THE BACK OF YOUR PARTNER'S RIGHT SHOULDER!

Dancing Don'ts

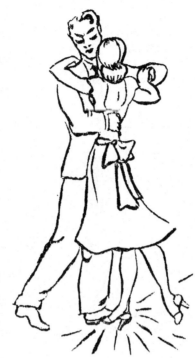

When left is left and
right is right,
the twain will
never meet!

DON'T start off on the wrong foot! The man always starts with his left foot—the girl with her right. Easy? Sure, if you know your left from your right . . . do you?

DON'T, girls, oh don't hang your full weight on your partner's arm . . . he can't dance for both of you. You're a big girl now—balance on your own two feet and support your own weight. If you can't, then stay home and take your vitamins.

DON'T, brother, don't walk forward all of the time. Your girl friend will get mighty tired of backing up all evening.

79

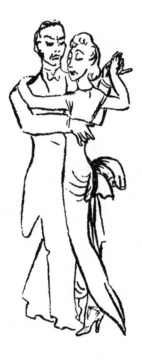

*Crabbing is a good sport—
for fishermen.
A smile makes better bait
for dancers.*

Try strolling backward for five minutes straight and you'll get the idea.

DON'T criticize your partner's dancing . . . this goes for both sexes. Finding fault with the other fellow is a sure sign of a beginner—or worse, of a sourpuss.

DON'T, little lady, blame your crushed toe on your partner. Maybe your back steps are too short. Test yourself—are the toes of your new slippers soiled already? Then, practice long steps, stretching back with your toes. Get out of his way!

DON'T be a sad-eyed Sammy or a sour-apple Sue. The

80

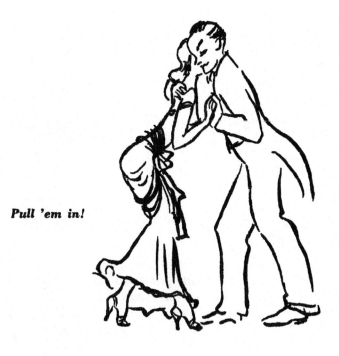

Pull 'em in!

dance floor is a place for fun . . . do your worrying on your own time. Smile now . . . or you're apt to have no one to smile with.

DON'T, girls, believe for a minute that all you have to do is relax. To relax is to collapse. Be alert, full of pep, on your toes—then you'll be fun to dance with!

DON'T forget that the best position for dancing is the same as for walking—keep erect. Dancing with hips 'way back is out-of-date. Besides, remember the stag line's view . . . you owe something to your public!

81

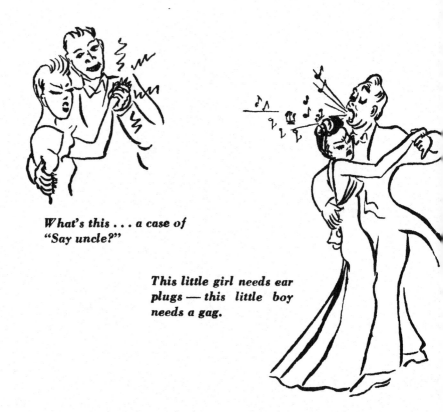

What's this . . . a case of "Say uncle?"

This little girl needs ear plugs — this little boy needs a gag.

DON'T clutch your partner's hand too firmly. You may not know your own strength! And, girls, don't take a death grip on the poor man's thumb . . . you've got him safely hooked for the dance—he can't get away.

DON'T hum or sing loudly—you're only an inch from your partner's ear. Humming or singing is fine if you're good enough to compete with the orchestra. But if you aren't sure of the tune or the words, do your warbling in the shower. Soaping and singing make a swell duet.

82

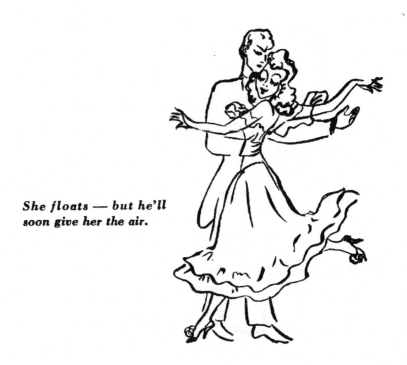

*She floats — but he'll
soon give her the air.*

DON'T be a butterfly, little girl. You have arms, not wings. A loose hold will make you miss the lead and stumble. What a comedown that will be! Hold your left hand in a firm grip on the back of your partner's shoulder . . . you'll keep your balance and your partner's praise.

DON'T hug the floor! LIFT YOUR FEET! Lift your feet a fraction of an inch off the floor and move through the air. Air offers no resistance—therefore, you can step lightly and effortlessly. Lift your feet slightly for graceful dancing.

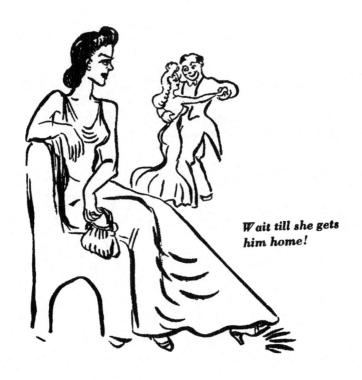

Wait till she gets him home!

DON'T keep apologizing. When you make a mistake, say "I'm sorry"—but just say it once. If you protest: "Gee, I'm clumsy" too often—someone may believe you.

DON'T expect a happy home life if you dance once with your wife—and then park her for the evening. You know what happens when cars are parked too long . . . they get cold; they gag and splutter, their carburetors overflow and their feed-lines don't work right for a long, long time.

Married couples shouldn't dance together for the whole

84

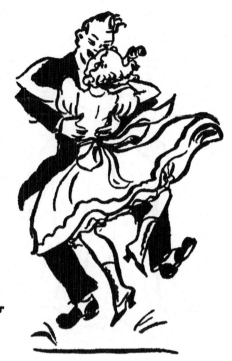

*The Polka was the
choice of sights
Careful ladies wore their
tights.*

evening. But, the way to do it gracefully is to change partners
with another couple. Four divides into two-and-two . . . a
much better combination than three.

DON'T go to extremes. A stately tread belongs in marble
halls . . . bouncing high is for the village green. They are both
too exaggerated for present day dancing.

Dancers used to hop high in the days of the Galop, Polka
and Leaping Waltz. Then, fashions changed and swung far
the other way. Dancing became overly conservative, dignified.

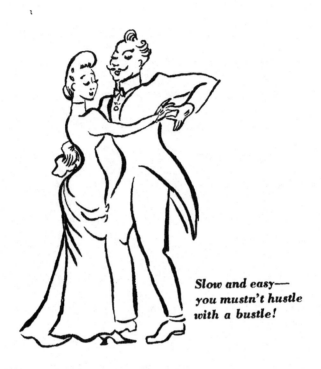

Slow and easy—
you mustn't hustle
with a bustle!

Every step seemed meticulously measured.

With this vogue for dignity—in about 1900—came the theory that good dancers must not lift their feet. Dancing teachers of the day preached: "Do not permit a crack of light to show between your feet and the floor."

This certainly made dull dancing. How can you dance lightly, with expression and animation, when your feet scrape the floor? Yet, even today, some pupils look surprised and skeptical when I tell them they must lift their feet while dancing.

Exercises to Improve Your Dancing

Aᴛ every newsstand you will find books of instructions for playing tennis, golf, swimming and so on. This information is easy to read and digest—but do you feel that you could perform these muscular activities just by knowing about them?

Dancing deals with the muscles, too. You can pick up steps just by watching them—or reading their description . . . but you will have your knowledge in your head only. Your feet and your body cannot respond to your will and desire alone—your muscles must first be trained to obey your command.

Men who want to be good dancers must learn only their own part—and train their muscles to follow the steps they choose to do. But girls are in a different position . . . they must be able to follow many partners—some tall, some short; some with a great variety of intricate steps, some with a weak lead and faltering steps.

The way to become an alert, agile partner—ready to follow anyone, is to train your muscles to obey quickly and to strengthen them to support you in any direction you choose to move.

You cannot dance merely by wanting to—any more than you can be a fine tennis player just because you know the rules and know that the game is fun to play.

To exercise sufficiently takes character and determination. It takes enthusiasm, too. If you really want to be a far better than average dancer—one who is sought out as a partner—you will study these exercises carefully. They are a sure means of training your dancing muscles quickly and effectively. Remember, no one can do it for you . . . but once you've achieved your ambition to be an attractive, popular partner—everyone will envy you.

Here are eight exercises for your use—you will find it more entertaining to do them in front of your mirror, in time with music.

EXERCISE 1

HAVE you ever wondered why some girls look better standing than others do? Or, have you ever wished that you knew how to stand when someone takes your snapshot?

Count One of this exercise will give you the same standing posture that the best photographers' models use. Count Two will give you the backstep technique of an exhibition dancer.

To make your feet look well as you stand, train your heels to always come together—as in the illustration. The toes should be turned out and the knees should touch each other. Look in your mirror!

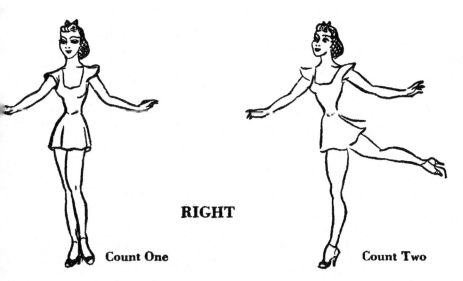

RIGHT

Count One   Count Two

On the count of One, bring your heels together so that your knees touch and your toes point outward. Now, on the count of Two, kick your right foot as far back as possible—toe pointed out and leading. Return to correct position of Count One. Repeat this same movement with your left foot and continue in time to slow Fox Trot music.

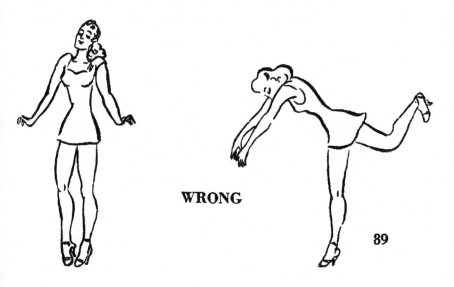

WRONG

89

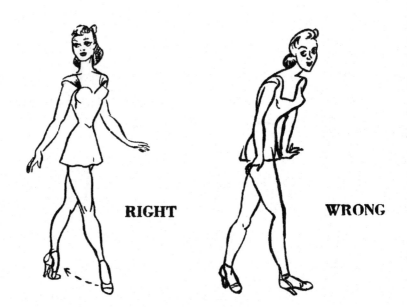

RIGHT　　　　　　　　**WRONG**

EXERCISE 2

This is an exercise that will train your feet and ankles to look attractive from any angle. It will teach you to automatically turn your toes outward—a definite "must" for any girl who wants to look well while dancing.

Place your feet together as in Exercise 1. Take a peek in your mirror to see how you're doing. Then, step backward with your left foot, counting One—draw your right foot up to your left, counting Two.

Now try the same thing with your right foot back.

Repeat this movement, going backward around the room. Don't forget that your toes must be turned outward.

This back step may seem exaggerated to you . . . but remember that most of your partners are going to walk you backward very often. You must prepare your muscles to carry you easily.

90

EXERCISE 3

THE illustration shows the finished product of this exercise. If you find it difficult to keep your balance, don't be discouraged—it merely proves that you need the practice. It will come easily after a few trys.

This is glamour training—it will develop supple muscles in your diaphragm and waistline.

Stand with your heels together, and your hands held loosely at your sides.

Step sideways on your right foot to the right, and draw your left foot behind the right, as you see in the correct illustration. At the same time, bring your arms and hands up in the position shown. Sway to the right.

Then step with your left foot to the left and bring your right foot up to and in back of your left. Sway to the left.

It is helpful to practice this to slow Waltz music, using three counts for each swaying movement. 1, 2, 3 to right; 4, 5, 6 to left.

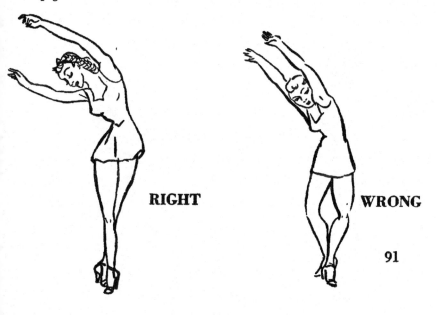

RIGHT   **WRONG**

EXERCISE 4

WHEN you first try this exercise, you may feel insecure. If so, lean on the top of your dresser or on the back of a chair until you can hold your balance.

This movement will train you to hold your head up high and it will gracefully arch your back. A stiff, unyielding back makes a girl feel wooden to her partner.

Begin by standing erect, with your hands at your sides and your heels together. Then swing into the position shown in the correct illustration.

Repeat, swinging back on the other foot.

This can be practiced to slow Waltz music or by counting 1, 2, 3. Don't bring your feet together again until after the third beat.

Note that the toes of the back-swinging foot are leading—and pointed outward.

CAUTION: Do not repeat these exercises too often the first time—or you will regret it the next day!

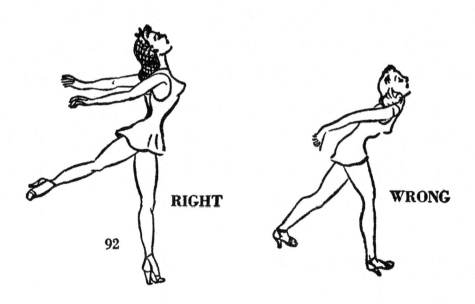

RIGHT   WRONG

92

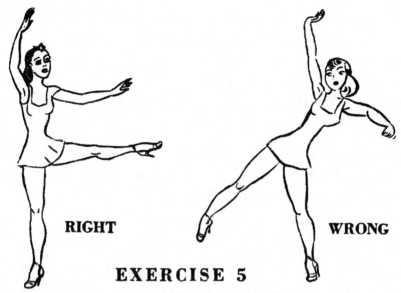

RIGHT   **WRONG**

EXERCISE 5

IF YOU can do this exercise correctly, with your body erect, you will develop a good sense of equilibrium. Practice it until you are well satisfied with your appearance in your mirror.

Simply extend one foot to the side and raise it as high as possible as shown in the illustration. Note that—again—your toes should lead.

Practice this ten times with one foot and then repeat to the other side.

When you have mastered this, with good balance and keeping your body erect, then rise on the toes of the foot carrying the weight.

Count: 1, 2, 3, 4. Raise foot 1, 2. Lower foot 3, 4. Try it to slow Fox Trot music.

This exercise will not only train you in balancing, but it will enable you to follow any quick side step that a partner may take.

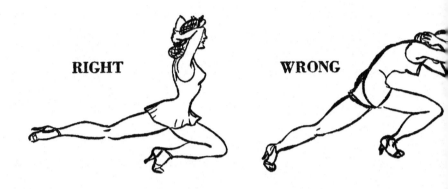

RIGHT   **WRONG**

EXERCISE 6

Do YOUR knees crra-ack as you bend? You can oil them with this exercise—it's meant to overcome stiff knee joints. It will help you to take smooth dancing steps, rather than the jerky movements of a beginner.

To begin: stand up straight in a natural position.

Take a long forward step with your right foot and place the weight on that foot. Bend the right knee and keeping your body erect, bend as far down as possible.

Not so easy? The results will be worth it—try again.

After bending, rise and resume your standing position. Now, without moving out of place, step forward with your left foot—weight on that foot—and bend as before.

Do this exercise gradually, a few times a day at first or you may need rubbing oil for your knees!

If you are practicing to music, allow three beats of a Waltz for the downward bend and three beats to rise to place.

94

EXERCISE 7

GIRLS who are not good dancers always dread dancing forward, toward their partners. It makes them feel insecure, clumsy—and they are in fear of stumbling over the man's feet.

Good dancers must be able to glide forward easily. In the Waltz, for instance, almost half the girl's steps will be toward her partner. This exercise will give you the security and confidence that you need; practice it.

Without bending your body forward, raise your right foot until it is parallel with the floor. Stretch your toes out—not up.

To develop dancing poise, hold your foot up for about five seconds, then lower it slowly. Repeat ten times, then try it with the other foot.

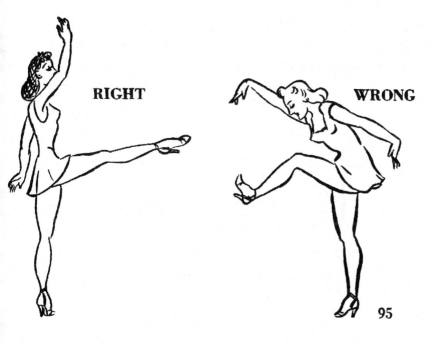

RIGHT

WRONG

95

EXERCISE 8

IT PUZZLES a man when he finds that some big, stout girls are easy and light to lead—while a slender 100 pounder may be as heavy as lead.

If you want to hear a man say to you: "You're wonderful to dance with—you're as light as a feather" . . . then train your arms. This exercise will do it—and further, it will add to your balance and poise.

Rise up on your right toe, raising your left leg backward, as high as you can. Let your toes lead and point outward. At the same time, bring your right arm up in the position shown in the picture. Hold this graceful pose for three beats of a Waltz measure, then slowly lower your hands and feet.

IMPORTANT! . . . Always make your wrists lead when using your arms and hands.

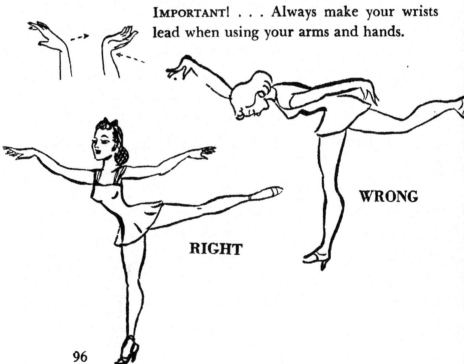

RIGHT

WRONG

96

Express Your Personality in Your Dancing

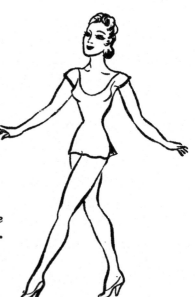

Read the rule of the "Law of Opposites".

In a whole roomful of dancers, did you ever spot one person whom you wished could be your partner? You'll notice that it isn't appearance alone that attracts you. There is another quality that draws your attention like a magnet. Call it "charm"—or "personality" . . . however you describe it, it shows in everything you do.

You can develop that extra something that will make your dancing personality colorful, attractive. It's easy, once you know the tricks that will do it.

First of all, accent your dancing! Give it highlights. Accent in dancing is a great deal like accent in speaking. A person who talks in a flat, level, unvarying voice is a bore to listeners. He may know a great deal and have a fine vocabu-

97

lary at his command but it all goes to waste because of his dreary, droning voice.

A man may know a great variety of steps and yet be a dull dancing partner. He must learn to accent his dancing to give it life and pep. Girls, too, must accent the beat and rhythm of the music before they can dance with expression.

To accent in dancing, merely emphasize the same beat of the music that the orchestra does. You can find this most easily by listening for the bass drum beats. Turn on your radio or phonograph and listen. Note that in a Waltz, the drummer strikes in measures of three beats but that he strikes hardest on each *first* beat.

Practice the Waltz, accenting or emphasizing the first of every three steps. Because a man always starts dancing with his left foot, his first accented step in the Waltz will be taken with his left. A girl will start accenting with her right foot.

It will take a few hours of practice before you can do this easily and automatically. But, it's worth the time—it will make dancing more fun for you, more exciting to your partners and more attractive to onlookers.

The Law of Opposites

Here is a secret of showmanship that will help you to express a sophisticated, smooth dancing personality. I call it the "Law of Opposites" and it is a rule that is used by every good dancer.

When you step forward with either foot, bring your opposite shoulder slightly forward. Look at the picture—note that the girl is stepping forward on her left foot and is turning her right shoulder slightly forward.

Try this movement of the body, while walking toward your mirror. It will remind you of the graceful, controlled steps that a high-diver takes on a springboard. Follow the rule of opposites in your dancing—it gives strength and assurance to the personality that you show.

The Face Must Dance, Too!

No dancer can attract partners by body and foot motion alone. The face must dance, too. Remember this—you are not dressed for dancing until you put on a smile! Show the cheerful side of your character when you dance—it will be contagious to your partner and to everyone who watches. Let them say of you . . . "What a wonderful personality!"

Do You Want People to Like You?

- Don't give helpful pointers while dancing. It makes you sound fault-finding.

- Don't steer your partner around the floor like a bicycle.

- Don't dance side-saddle.

- Don't chew gum in time to music. Don't chew gum in your partner's ear. Maybe . . . don't chew gum!

- Don't be so serious. Leave your business face at the office when you step out.

- Don't say you *hate* dancing just because you don't know how.

- If you want to lead a man to the altar—don't lead him on the dance floor.

- Don't let old-fashioned dancing date you!

- When you make a misstep, don't blame the orchestra.

- Don't brag "I never had a lesson in my life."

- Don't keep on dancing for "politeness' sake" when neither of you is having fun.

- Don't dance passively—be glad you're alive.

100

Etiquette of the Ballroom

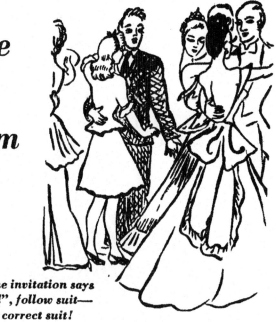

When the invitation says
"Formal", follow suit—
with the correct suit!

MANY people seem to shy away from the word "etiquette." It has an old-fashioned sound. But etiquette, after all, is merely the practical application of good common sense and attractive manners.

Ballroom dancing is a partnership and group activity and so it concerns other people beside yourself. There is never any excuse for faulty manners that might affect or react on others. A popular member of a dancing group is considerate—and shows regard for the comfort and pleasure of partners, a hostess and the other guests.

Once you have accepted an invitation to a dance, you have automatically agreed to live up to the obligations it

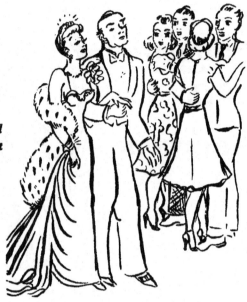

Too formal is bad form, too, if it is not requested.

implies. You are expected to be suitably dressed, to be pleasant company and, above all, to be able to dance.

No one would dream of accepting an invitation for tennis or bridge unless he could play. But many will accept dancing dates when they know quite well that their dancing is not good enough for a partner to enjoy. It's odd, isn't it?

If you can't dance with confidence, have the courage to refuse dancing invitations. Wait until you have the ability and can appear in the best light possible. By starting to practice immediately, you'll be ready and in demand the next time!

A man who accepts an invitation to a dance cannot spend the entire evening with the one partner of his choice. By accepting, he has agreed to add to the festivity of the evening

102

by mingling with the group, by asking several partners to dance or by changing partners with other couples. Natural courtesy dictates the rule that he must seek out and invite his hostess to dance. If she has daughters or sisters present, they must not be overlooked.

A girl must wait to be asked to dance, but she has her obligations to the party. She cannot, for instance, refuse one partner and then turn around and accept another. Neither should a girl attempt to tie strings to a partner—to hold on to him. She must release him gracefully so that he can get about and dance with others.

When entering or leaving the dance room, the girl always precedes. Men never go first unless they need to do so to give assistance, such as in helping a girl out of a car, bus or so on.

It is no longer considered good taste for a man to take the girl's arm when they are walking to or from the dance floor. This has been out-of-date for years.

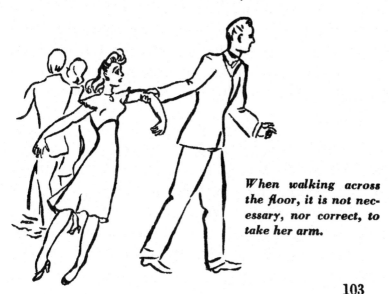

When walking across the floor, it is not necessary, nor correct, to take her arm.

103

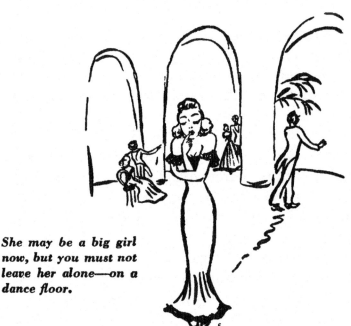

She may be a big girl now, but you must not leave her alone—on a dance floor.

There is a right and wrong way to ask a girl to dance. It puts her in an awkward spot if you say: "Have you the next dance taken?" What girl wants to admit that her dances are not taken! Instead, say: "May I have the next dance?" Don't forget this . . . it holds true for all invitations. It is more polite to say: "Will you go dancing with me on Friday night?" . . . than to tactlessly say: "What are you doing on Friday night?" See the difference?

At the end of each dance, a man must always escort his partner back to where she was sitting. He must never leave her in the middle of the floor. But don't forget, he doesn't have to take her by the arm to lead her off!

When leaving a girl after dancing with her, a man should make some pleasant remark like: "Thank you so much—I enjoyed dancing with you." He should be careful not to say:

104

"I'll be back later," unless he plans to return. A man is well protected by the rules of etiquette. If he has had an uncongenial or dull partner, he can make his exit very smoothly by saying that he must find the girl with whom he has the next dance. Or, that he has not yet danced with the hostess.

Cutting-in

This is an acceptable custom at almost all dances that are held in America. If a man wants to cut-in on the girl of his choice, he should wait until she is dancing fairly near him, at the outer edge of the floor. Then he can easily step to her side and nod pleasantly, saying "May I?" to her partner.

It is considered childishly bad form to refuse to "break." Instead, the man who has been cut-in on, should step aside good-naturedly, with a slight bow and a smile, and join the stag line. From there, he can do a little cutting-in himself.

There is a generally accepted rule that there must be an

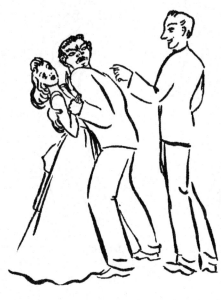

A cut-in is legal; you may be giving up your partner reluctantly, but do it cheerfully.

105

intervening cut-in before a man can return to claim his original partner. For instance, if Bill cuts-in on John ... John should not cut back on Bill. He should wait until another man is dancing with the girl.

The cut-in system is very cruel to a girl. Even when she likes the partner she has, she yearns for cut-ins, to prove her popularity. But, no matter how welcome the "cut" is, a girl should not show undue glee. She should smile equally at her original partner and at her new one.

A girl who pounces on a new cut-in with obvious delight makes him wary and suspicious. Further, her stock goes down with a bang because she has been noticeably insulting to her original partner. Neither can she show reluctance to break,

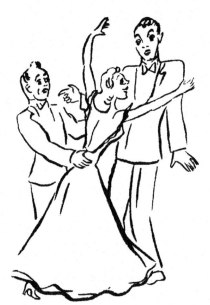

Take it easy, sister, smile to the old before welcoming the new!

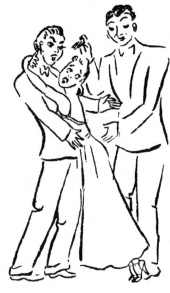

Cut-ins are a sign of popularity — welcome them. Besides, it's rude to refuse.

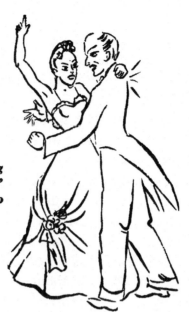

Debating and dancing both begin with a "d"—but they don't go together.

even when her original partner is her dream man. Girls must chart their course very carefully for smooth sailing.

Conversation

This is a matter of personality but there are general rules of good manners to consider. The first taboo is don't argue! Dancing is a partnership that depends on accord. Two people cannot move as one and enjoy the rhythm of the music together unless they feel harmonious toward each other. So, avoid subjects that might breed discord; such as politics, religion, school elections and so on. Even when you discuss songs or bands, remember that the sweetest words ever spoken are: "I think you're right!"

There are some people who cannot talk as they dance. Theirs is a companionable silence because it is obvious that their minds are occupied with the rhythm of the music and the pleasure of the dance.

The strong, stern, silent man and the frosty-faced, forbidding female don't belong at a dance. Their partners find them unpleasant and the onlookers will avoid them. There may be some reason not to talk as you dance . . . but always keep your smile on!

The walkie-talkie chatter-box is a conversational hazard, too. There are always a few at every dance . . . they are so keyed up or so shy that they have forgotten all about Silence Being Golden. Their chatter is so steady that it drowns out the loudest band. Like the brook, they ripple on and on. Nothing can be done about it but you can profit by their example!

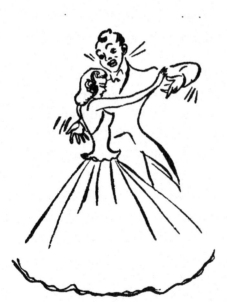

If you can't talk and dance at the same time, just dance.

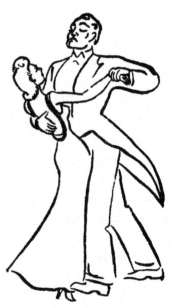

If you're the strong, silent type, do it with a smile.

Introductions

Introducing people is a bugbear to those who are shy . . .
and to those who are young and unpracticed. Actually, the
only difficult part is to remember names—and to have them
at the tip of your tongue. Otherwise, your cues are easy . . .
you always present the man to the girl, mentioning her name
first. Such as: "Lillian, this is Mr. Brown—Miss Smith." Or,
if you are not on first-name terms with her, you can say:
"Miss Smith, may I present Mr. Brown."

When introducing two women, you present the younger
one to the older, such as: "Mrs. Jones, this is Miss Smith."
If they are of equal age, it doesn't matter which name is men-
tioned first. "Mrs. Jones, I'd like to have you know Mrs.
Brown."

Acknowledging Introductions

It is good training to make a point of remembering
names; therefore many people form the habit of acknowledg-
ing introductions by repeating the name. Such as: "How do
you do, Mrs. Brown." If you have not really heard the other
person's name, it will flatter them to have you say: "Did you
say Mrs. Brown? . . . How do you do."

Don't make the famous mistake that was made by a
young girl, who was too shy to ask to have the name repeated
—and who, later in the evening, asked: "I'm not quite sure—
how do you spell your name?" "S-M-I-T-H, plain Smith," he
replied.

Certain replies to introductions have fallen into too
common usage and are not considered good taste. As an

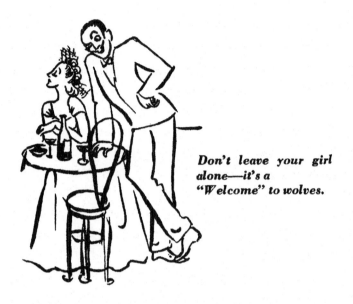

Don't leave your girl alone—it's a "Welcome" to wolves.

example: "Pleased to meet you" . . . is no longer used. Yet, "I'm so glad to know you" is quite acceptable.

A woman does not rise to acknowledge introductions, unless she is the hostess, or is being introduced to an older person. A hostess rises to greet all of her guests, men or women.

Night Club Dancing

So far, we have discussed private dancing parties.

A restaurant, featuring dancing, is quite different. Here your only obligation is to the people of your own party. A cut-in from a stranger should never be accepted . . . nor should it be offered. A man should avoid leaving his date alone at the table unless it is really necessary. Otherwise, she may be subjected to unwelcome attention.

Most restaurant and night club dance floors are tiny in

size. So, in consideration of your partner and your neighbors, you should avoid complicated steps. Dance simply and follow the line of direction. This means to progress around the room, clockwise. Shorten your steps to fit the limitation of space.

One Last Word

It is not bad manners to suggest sitting down before the dance is over. That is, if you suggest the idea tactfully. Either partner can say: "It's warm in here, don't you think so? Shall we sit out and cool off for a few moments?" Or, "It's crowded, isn't it? I'm anxious to talk to you anyway — shall we sit down?"

From now on, try to think more kindly of the word "etiquette"—it protects you, too; don't you think so?

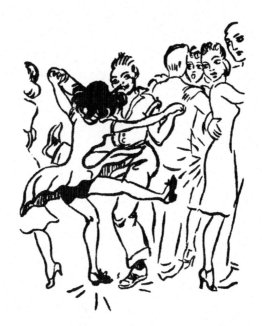

Exhibition dancing needs an empty floor and a willing audience.

CPSIA information can be obtained at www.ICGtesting.com
Printed in the USA
BVOW08s0221290515

402008BV00010B/305/P